THE DIETING GUIDE FOR LYMPHATIC SYSTEM

A Comprehensive Cookbook to Manage Common Lymphatic Disease

Copyright @ 2023 by **BREN HAN PHD**

TABLE OF CONTENT

INTRODUCTION

Lymph is a clear fluid which collects and carries proteins, fats, bacteria, excess fluid and damaged cells around the body via tube-like structures called lymph vessels. Lymph fluid is transported to lymph nodes where the fluid is routinely processed and cleaned by immune cells also known as white blood cells. Think back to the last time you were fighting a cold or felt run down. Do you remember feeling small, tender bumps around the sides your neck?

Those lumps were probably swollen lymph nodes; the sign of a normal and healthy immune response! When we are under the weather, lymph nodes spring into action and begin fighting off pathogens and other foreign particles. Once this job is done, the lymphatic system returns to business as usual; clearing toxins and waste from the body's tissues.

With approximately 700 lymph nodes spread throughout the human body, it's no wonder the lymphatic system has a strong influence on our overall health. Firstly, the lymphatic system helps to maintain fluid balance in the body.

When the lymphatic system is under pressure and stress, the volume of fluid surrounding bodily tissue can increase which results in fluid retention and swelling. It is the job of healthy lymph capillaries to reduce excess fluid and restore balance in the body.

Secondly, it has been highlighted that lymphatic system is important for the absorption of dietary fats and fat-soluble vitamins in the digestive system. Thirdly, and probably the most well-known function of the lymphatic system, is it's defense against disease and invading microorganisms. As such, the lymphatic system is thought to be involved in a variety of health conditions from infections to cancer to metabolic and inflammatory diseases.

To summarized this know that the lymphatic system helps in detoxification of waste products from the body, Immunity boosts to keep the body healthy and Transportation of nutrients throughout the body.

First and foremost, the lymphatic system works as sort of a trash collector and disposal system. It pumps lymphatic fluids throughout the body and absorbs toxins, wastes, and other nasty stuff and then helps eliminate it from the body.

Without proper lymphatic systems performing its detoxification, toxins would quickly accumulate and cause major problems with every major organ and system in the body and ultimately it would lead to organ failure and tissue death. The lymphatic system also absorbs fats and important vitamins and spreads them throughout the body to the areas they are needed and thus helps keep nutrient levels balanced.

One of the major components of the lymph system is the thymus and the bone marrow. These two systems are very important in the production of antibodies, regenerative cells, and work to help identify invading viruses and bacteria and helps the body fight off illness and disease. The healthy function of these two systems is enhanced greatly by appropriate lymph circulation, good hydration, and a proper pH balance in the body. The importance of the lymphatic system is easily seen when it comes to the immune system and protecting the body against illnesses and boosting the body's ability to stay healthy and strong.

Even though the lymph system is a type of circulatory system, it does not have a pump like the heart functions for blood circulation.

Instead, the lymph system uses lymph vessels and lymph nodes to absorb the fluids and utilizes the pumping movement of the bones and muscles as we move to push the fluids throughout the body. Being active and moving is critical to the lymph system functioning at maximum efficiency. Without the squeezing of the lymphatic vessels by muscles all the toxins and waste materials begin to accumulate in tissue and this causes pain and inflammation and can lead to illness and a host of other problems.

CHAPTER ONE

COMMON DISEASES OF LYMPHATIC SYSTEM

There are several conditions that can affect the lymph vessels, lymph nodes, and lymphatic organs. The three most common lymphatic diseases include:

Lymphadenopathy is the medical term for swollen or enlarged lymph nodes. It can occur due to inflammation, infection, or cancer. When the cause of a swollen lymph node is infections or inflammatory disorders, it is called lymphadenitis. For example, strep throat can cause enlargement of regional lymph nodes in the neck. Breast cancer can lead to enlarged lymph nodes in the axillae (armpits).

Lymphedema: This medical term refers to a buildup of lymphatic fluid in the tissues. It most commonly occurs in the arms and legs. Lymphatic system blockages can cause lymphedema due to scar tissue, tumors, or damaged lymph nodes or lymph vessels. Lymphedema can also occur when lymph nodes are surgically removed or subjected to radiation during cancer treatment.

Severe lymphedema can be painful, disabling, and disfiguring and can put a person at risk of serious infections.

When lymphocytes (white blood cells) multiply uncontrolled, it can result in a cancer called lymphoma. Two common types of lymphoma are Hodgkin lymphoma and non-Hodgkin lymphoma.

Some other disorders that can affect the body's lymphatic system include:

- Tonsillitis: An infection and inflammation of the tonsils in the throat.

- Lymphangitis: An inflammation of the lymphatic vessels.

- Lymphocytosis: The presence of too many white blood cells.

- Mesenteric lymphadenitis: An inflammation of lymph nodes in the mesentery (an organ attached to the intestines in the abdomen).

- Lymphatic filariasis: A parasitic infection of the lymphatic system that leads to massive swelling in the arms, legs, and genitals.

- Intestinal lymphangiectasia: A condition in which lymph is lost in the small intestine, leading to protein loss.

MANAGING YOUR LYMPHATIC SYSTEM WITH LYMPHATIC DRAINAGE

Lymphatic drainage massage has been trending in recent years, with celebrities and health personalities alike claiming it can help flush out toxins, give your immune system a boost and even help you shed unwanted pounds. But is it legit? And who can benefit? Lymphatic drainage massage is a gentle massage that targets the lymphatic system, which resides just beneath the skin. It is powerful tool for people whose lymphatic system is compromised from surgery, illness or injury. But unfortunately, lymphatic drainage is often misunderstood.

How? The lymphatic system is a network of vessels and organs that lie beneath the skin, and it's a critical component of a healthy immune system. In fact, your lymphatic system acts almost like a garbage disposal, helping your body filter out waste and bacteria.

Lymphatic drainage massage, which is sometimes called manual lymphatic drainage, or MLD, involves gently massaging areas of the body to help move lymph fluid to an area with working lymph vessels.

Normally, the lymphatic system collects lymph fluid and returns it to your heart through the lymph vessels and nodes. But when there's a disruption to your lymphatic system's process, such as the removal of lymph nodes during surgery for breast cancer, the fluid can collect in your arms and legs, which leads to swelling. The medical term for swelling is edema, so the condition is called lymphedema.

Some certified therapists commonly use MLD to relieve swelling by coaxing lymph fluid from your tissues to your functioning lymph nodes. Unlike traditional massage, lymphatic drainage massage uses light pressure to mobilize the lymphatic system, which lies directly beneath the skin.

MLD follows a specific sequence, starting with the main drains in the body, including the lymph nodes in the neck, groin and armpits. The idea is that by massaging an area where there is no swelling, the congested lymph fluid will have somewhere to go because you've created space for it.

Would you benefit from Lymphatic Massage? All our cells rely on lymph fluid to boost immunity and transport waste products. So theoretically, a congested lymphatic system can compromise your immune system. And since lymph fluid is full of disease-fighting white blood cells, stuck fluid can contribute to a host of issues, including lymphedema. The most obvious sign of a compromised lymphatic system is swelling. Like the blood that's part of your circulatory system, lymph fluid is constantly moving.

If it stops, lymph fluid can build up and create swelling, usually in the arms and legs. If your rings feel tight or your clothes begin to feel a bit snugger, that could be a sign that you're holding on to excess fluid. You might also experience pain and a feeling of heaviness.

Most of the time, lymphatic vessels become congested as a result of surgery, infection, trauma or diseases like cancer.

So, chances are good that if your lymphatic system is suffering, you'd know it. Infection and tight muscles may also be signs of congestion.

In addition to cancer, conditions such as rheumatoid arthritis, fibromyalgia, chronic venous insufficiency (which happens when your leg veins aren't working correctly) and lipedema (where abnormal fat accumulates in your body) can cause lymphedema.

Also, if you have a healthy lymphatic system, lymphatic drainage massage isn't likely to benefit you beyond simple relaxation.

And despite celebrities claiming that lymphatic drainage massage makes them red-carpet ready, there's no evidence that lymphatic drainage massage can help you slim down.

Instead, using lymphatic drainage techniques may have a temporary trimming effect because it helps move fluid through the body (like spreading a stack of papers from one end of the counter across the entire surface).

Types of Lymphatic Drainage Massage

Manual lymphatic drainage is a professional massage performed by trained specialists. Massage therapists usually use the following MLD techniques:

Vodder: This method was named after Dr. Vodder, who studied swollen lymph nodes and developed the manual lymphatic drainage technique. It involves massaging the patient using four basic movements: sweeping motions, stationary circles, pumping movements, and rotary movements.

Foldi: This technique is an extension of the Vodder method. It involves alternating between massaging the patient and moments of relaxation, including deep breathing.

Casley-Smith: In this technique, the therapist mainly uses the sides and palms of the hands, massaging the patient in slow, repetitive, circular motions. The method often incorporates compression bandaging as part of the treatment protocol.

> Leduc: Involves making slow, circular movements in a single direction to improve lymphatic flow. The technique often combines lymphatic drainage with other massage elements, such as deep tissue massage and myofascial release.

A manual lymphatic drainage massage typically takes 30-60 minutes.

Lymphatic Drainage Massage Benefits

Helps Relieve Symptoms of Certain Medical Conditions

Drainage massage is often used to treat lymphedema patients. This condition is characterized by the swelling of arms and legs due to cancer treatments, surgery, genetic disorders, infection, and injury. The massage may also help relieve swelling, pain, and stiffness in patients with rheumatoid arthritis, fibromyalgia, lipedema, and chronic venous insufficiency.

Improves Circulation

Lymphatic drainage massage indirectly improves circulation by removing toxins and waste products from tissues and by reducing swelling, which can restrict blood flow.

Increases Relaxation and Alleviates Stress

Lymphatic drainage involves gentle, rhythmic motions close to the skin's surface that ease muscle tension and promote calmness. Studies also show that massage stimulates the parasympathetic nervous system, which reduces stress and tension and helps patients relax.

May Stimulate the Immune System

Lymphatic drainage massage reroutes blocked lymph to healthy lymph nodes, helping filter toxins, waste, and pathogens. Eliminating harmful substances may reduce the risk of infections and illness, improving immune function.

May Help with Skin Conditions

Trapped lymph around and above the neck containing toxins, debris, and inflammatory cells often causes skin conditions such as acne, edema, eczema, and psoriasis. Lymphatic drainage massage moves the lymph and inflammatory cells down, below the neck, clearing problematic facial skin.

May Help Rejuvenate the Skin

Removing excess fluid with a facial lymphatic drainage massage may help reduce swelling, lift and tighten the skin, and temporarily rejuvenate the face.

May Improve Cellulite

By reducing fluid retention and swelling, lymphatic drainage massage reduces the amount of fluid pressing against the fibers beneath the skin. It can help improve the appearance of cellulite.

How Do you Know if you Need Lymphatic Drainage?

You can benefit from lymphatic drainage if you notice the following symptoms:

Swelling in the arms and legs

Swollen lymph nodes

Stiff joints

Muscle pain

Depression

Constant tiredness

Bloating

Problems with digestion

Constipation

Brain fog

Dull, dry, or itchy skin

Allergies

Some of these symptoms can also be signs of more serious conditions so make sure you consult your physician before scheduling a lymphatic drainage massage.

How to Prepare for Lymphatic Drainage Massage

The following tips will help you prepare for lymphatic drainage massage and reduce the risk of side effects.

• Drink plenty of water before (and after) the massage to encourage lymph flow.

• Eat a light meal before the treatment.

• Don't take ibuprofen and other blood thinners one week before the massage to reduce the risk of bruising.

• Wear loose, comfortable clothing to reduce discomfort and avoid impeding natural lymph flow.

CHAPTER TWO

DIETING FOR LYMPHATIC SYSTEMS

What you eat is an important part of both your physical and mental health. A well-balanced diet makes you feel good, simple as that! Eating healthy produces less waste for your lymphatic system to clean up, and avoiding this like processed foods that are high in salt, sugar, and preservatives will reduce your chances of lymphatic congestion. Natural foods like dark green vegetables, ginger, citrus fruits, flaxseed, and garlic are ideal for lymphatic cleansing.

Incorporating a regular detox cleanse that is supported by liver enzymes will ease the stress on your liver and kidneys, and lessen the amount of work your body has to do to get rid of toxins from what you eat.

The old adage you are what you eat couldn't be truer than when applied to your lymphatic health. We all know the importance of eating a healthy balanced diet, but are not aware of the role the lymphatic system plays in aiding the digestive process However, did you know that there are other foods that can actively help boost lymphatic flow?

It's not surprising that our lymphatic system, like the rest of our body, depends on a well-balanced diet rich in vitamins and minerals to keep it in peak condition. If our body is experiencing a high level of inflammation, this can put increased stress on the lymphatic system and overtime this can lead to dysfunction and impairment. To ensure that you are supporting the drainage and filtering power of the lymphatic system make sure to take in plenty of water and foods with anti-inflammatory properties and reduce your intake of foods that can increase inflammation within the body.

Different vegetables are packed with various enzymes and antioxidants that help the body combat and filter out the body's impurities with ease. Leafy green perform excellently in breaking down toxins; they possess chlorophyll, an essential detoxification agent that can aid the cleansing of blood vessels and lymph nodes. They facilitate lymph circulation which enables infections to be dealt with by the lymph nodes efficiently.

A lot of these leafy greens also come packed with water content, so they also provide optimum hydration. In particular we recommend, Kale, Spinach, Cabbage, Watercress, Romaine Lettuce, Swiss Chard and Bok Choi.

Plants, fruit and vegetables traditionally used to produce red dyes (cherries, berries, pomegranates, beetroot and cranberries) were frequently used in Ayurvedic and other Eastern medicines to boost lymphatic flow when signs of stagnation occurred. This is because the compounds responsible for their intense colour (such as anthocyanins, lycopene and betalain) are powerful antioxidants and anti-inflammatory agents. Research has also shown that anthocyanins are effective against cancer, ageing, neurological disease, chronic inflammation and diabetes.

To keep your lymph flowing freely, be sure to load up on lots of lovely red fruit and veg. Cherries, raspberries, red cabbage, pomegranate and beetroot are especially high in anthocyanins.

Deserving of particular attention are cranberries, which are great fat emulsifiers and will help break down excess fat for easier absorption and transportation through the lymphatic system.

Beets particularly beetroot help to thin the bile, which has been shown to play a major role in the immune response of the gut. Bile also regulates the stool, helps digest good fat and disposes of bad fat. Beets also scrub the villi of the gut, which is where digestive lymph originates in the lacteals.

One of the most powerful lymph-supporting red foods is the Manjistha root. Highly prized in Ayurvedic medicine for its ability to boost lymphatic flow and overall health. Manjistha (or Rubia cordifolia, meaning "red root") has been found to support the liver when it is exposed to high levels of toxins by boosting the production of glutathione, recognised as one of the body's most powerful anti-oxidants. Difficult to come by in it's fresh state, there are many Manjistha supplements that are available in powder and capsule form.

Including yellow foods in your diet can provide several benefits from healthy hearts and improved circulation to better immunity. Lemons are well known to cleanse toxins from any part of the body and Ayurvedic medicine uses both lemons and lemon essential oil to treat a significant number of health conditions.

Ginger has been used for centuries and is highly prized in Chinese medicine where it is regarded as a warming herb with particular benefits for the lymph nodes, spleen, heart and digestive organs.

A staple in India for thousands of years, turmeric is wonderful for increasing circulation and enhancing the detox function of the liver. It also increases the body's antioxidant levels, stimulates the metabolism and is a powerful anti-inflammatory.

Sweet potatoes are rich in antioxidants and have four times the recommended daily intake of Beta-Carotene, converted by the body into Vitamin A, which has a critical role to play in immune function.

Cottage Cheese with Fruit Breakfast Bowls

Total Time: 35 Minutes

INGREDIENTS

- ½ tablespoon lime zest ~1 small lime

- 3 tablespoons fresh lime juice ~½ lime

- 3 tablespoons honey

- 6 mint leaves thinly sliced

- 1 cup blueberries

- 1 cup sliced strawberries

- 1 lb. cottage cheese ~2 cups

DIRECTIONS

- Place the lime zest, juice, and honey into a bowl and whisk together. Add the mint leaves, blueberries, and strawberries and mix to coat with the dressing. Set aside.

- a white bowl with berries and blueberries in it.

- To serve, place ½ cup of cottage cheese into a bowl and top with ½ cup of the fresh berry mixture.

Smoked Salmon and Avocado Wraps

Total Time: 15 Minutes

INGREDIENTS

- 1 piece flat bread (see intro mountain bread)

- 100g smoked salmon

- 1 avocado

- 1 tablespoon mayonnaise

- 1 tablespoon dill (chopped)

- 1 tablespoon american mustard (I used Dijon mustard)

- 1 carrot (small shredded)

- 4 lettuce leaves (large)

- lemon juice (just a squeeze)

DIRECTIONS

- Mix together the avocado, dill, mayonnaise, mustard and lemon juice until all combined.

- Lay down 1 piece of mountain bread and smear with the avocado mixture, then top with the smoked salmon and shredded carrot and top off with the lettuce and then roll up the mountain bread nice and tight, wrap firmly with cling wrap and place in the fridge (overnight is great), cut into slices and serve.

Overnight Oats with Blueberries and Almonds

Total Time: 8 Hours 5 Minutes

INGREDIENTS

- ¾ cup old-fashioned oats

- ½ to ¾ cup milk (such as whole, skim, almond, soy or coconut)

- 1 tablespoon maple syrup

- ⅓ cup yogurt

- 3 tablespoons sliced almonds

- ¼ cup blueberries

DIRECTIONS

- Pour the oats into a 1-pint mason jar.

- In a small bowl, mix the milk with the maple syrup. (If you prefer a thicker oatmeal, use less milk.)

- Pour the milk mixture into the jar. Screw on the lid and refrigerate overnight, about 8 hours.

- In the morning, top the oatmeal with the yogurt, sliced almonds and blueberries. Eat immediately or screw the top on and take it on the go.

Quinoa Stuffed Peppers

Total Time: 55 Minutes

INGREDIENTS

- 6 medium bell peppers tops cut off and cores removed

- 1 cup uncooked quinoa rinsed and drained

- 2 cups vegetable broth

- 1 tablespoon olive oil

- 1 small onion chopped

- 2 garlic cloves minced

- 1 15 ounce canned diced tomatoes

- 1 15 ounce can black beans

- 1 cup frozen corn thawed

- 1 teaspoon cumin

- 1 teaspoon paprika

- ½ teaspoon salt

- ¼ teaspoon black pepper

- 1 cup freshly shredded Monterey Jack cheese

- Optional toppings: chopped fresh cilantro diced avocado, sour cream

DIRECTIONS

- Place the quinoa and vegetable broth in a medium saucepan. Bring the mixture to a boil over medium-high heat. Lower heat to a simmer, cover the saucepan with a lid and cook covered until all the liquid is absorbed, 15 minutes. Allow the quinoa to rest for about 5 minutes, without opening the lid, then fluff with a fork.

- Preheat oven to 375°F, and prepare the peppers by cutting them in half lengthwise and removing the seeds and membrane. Place the peppers in a baking dish cut side up, and pour water around the peppers just enough to cover the bottom of the pan.

- Heat olive oil in a large nonstick skillet over medium heat. Add onions and saute until they start to soften, about 2-3 minutes. Add the garlic and cook until fragrant, 1 more minute. Stir in the cooked quinoa, diced tomatoes, black beans and corn. Season with cumin, paprika, salt and pepper. Reduce heat to low and cook for additional 5 minutes, stirring frequently.

- Carefully spoon the mixture into the sliced peppers and sprinkle the cheese on top.

- Bake uncovered until the peppers are tender and the cheese is melted, about 30-35 minutes. Add optional toppings and serve hot.

Lemon Herb Grilled Chicken

Total Time: 1 Hour 15 Minutes

INGREDIENTS

- 2 lbs chicken breasts, trimmed

- 1/4 cup olive oil, extra virgin

- 1/4 cup lemon juice

- 1 tbsp dried basil

- 1 tbsp dried parsley

- 1 tsp salt

- 1/2 tsp black pepper

- 1/2 tsp garlic powder

- 1/2 tsp onion powder

- 1/4 tsp crushed red pepper flakes

DIRECTIONS

- Place your chicken breasts in a gallon Ziploc bag with all ingredients for the Lemon Herb Marinade. Seal the bag, squeezing out any excess air. Let the chicken marinate for at least one hour and up to 12 hours.

- Grill or saute your chicken depending on your preference. I'm providing instructions for both below.

<u>**TO GRILL**</u>

- Remove each chicken breast from the bag and place on a hot grill over medium heat. Grill 5 to 7 minutes on each side or until done. (Juices should run clear.)

ON THE STOVE

- Add 2 tablespoons of olive oil or another cooking fat to a skillet on the stove. Heat the oil over medium high heat. (You'll know it's ready when the chicken sizzles as you place it in the pan.) Add each chicken breast to the skillet in a single layer. Cook for about 5 minutes. Flip your chicken. Cook for an additional 5 minutes. (Chicken should be firm to the touch when done and juices should run clear.)

Quinoa Stir Fry with Vegetables

Total Time: 30 Minutes

Ingredients

- 1 cup uncooked quinoa

- ½ julienned onion

- ½ julienned red bell pepper

- 1 cup julienned red cabbage

- 1 julienned carrot

- ½ head of broccoli, chopped, discard the stem

- 2 tablespoon extra virgin olive oil

- 4 sliced cloves of garlic

- ¼ teaspoon cayenne powder

- ½ teaspoon ground ginger

- 1 tablespoon tamari or soy sauce

- 1 tablespoon cane or coconut sugar

- Sesame seeds

DIRECTIONS

- Cook the quinoa according to package directions. Read this post if you want to learn how to cook quinoa properly.

- Boil or steam the veggies for about 2 minutes. You want crunchy vegetables. Drain and set aside.

- Heat the oil in a wok or a frying pan and cook the garlic over medium-high heat for about a couple of minutes.

- Add the cayenne powder and the veggies and cook for another 2 minutes, stirring frequently.

- Add the quinoa and the rest of the ingredients (except the sesame seeds) and cook for 2 minutes more.

- Serve with some sesame seeds on top.

- Store in a sealed container in the fridge for about 5 days.

Turkey Meatballs over Zucchini Noodles

Total Time: 30 Minutes

Ingredients

- 1 lb. ground turkey

- 1/4 c. seasoned dry breadcrumbs

- 1 large egg

- 3 tbsp. chopped fresh flat-leaf parsley

- 1 1/2 oz. Parmesan cheese, grated (about 1/3 c.), plus more for serving

- 2 garlic cloves, chopped, divided

- Kosher salt

- Freshly ground black pepper

- 2 tbsp. extra-virgin olive oil, divided

- 1 (25-oz.) jar marinara sauce

- 4 medium zucchini, cut into noodles with a spiralizer or julienne peeler

- 4 oz. Provolone cheese, grated (about 1 c.)

DIRECTIONS

- Combine turkey, breadcrumbs, egg, parsley, Parmesan, 1 garlic clove, and 1/2 teaspoon each salt and pepper in a bowl. Form into 12 (1 1/2" to 2") meatballs.

- Heat 1 tablespoon oil in a large skillet over medium heat. Add meatballs and cook, turning occasionally, until brown on all sides, 4 to 6 minutes. Reduce heat to medium-low and gently stir in marinara. Simmer, turning meatballs occasionally, until meatballs are cooked through and sauce is thickened, 14 to 16 minutes.

- Meanwhile, heat remaining tablespoon oil in a medium skillet over medium-high heat. Add zucchini and remaining garlic and cook until just tender and heated through, 2 to 3 minutes. Season with salt and pepper.

- Heat broiler to high with rack in the top position. Sprinkle provolone over meatballs. Broil until cheese is golden brown, 3 to 4 minutes.

- Serve meatballs over noodles topped with Parmesan.

Crispy Turmeric Roasted Chickpeas

Total Time: 40 Minutes

Ingredients

- 400 grams canned chickpeas

- 3 tbs olive oil

- 1 ts red paprika

- ½ ts turmeric

- cayenne pepper

- salt

- ginger

- thyme, oregano

Directions

- Preheat oven to 200°C / 390°F.

- Drain chickpeas, wash and thoroughly dry. If any skin comes off, you can remove it, but this is optional. Use paper towels to completely dry your chickpeas.

- In a bowl, pour olive oil, then add your spices: 1 ts red paprika, 1/2 ts turmeric, a pinch of cayenne pepper, a pinch of salt, a pinch of ginger, thyme and oregano. Combine well.

- Add dried chickpeas to the olive oil coating and toss to combine.

- Place coated chickpeas on a baking tray, lined with baking paper or aluminium foil and bake for about 30 minutes, or until the chickpeas turn golden-brown. Remove from oven and set aside to cool. During cooling, the chickpeas will turn crispy. Serve as snack, or as topping in soups or salads.

Fried Brown Rice with Shrimp and Snap Peas

Ingredients

- 1 ½ (8.8-ounce) pouches precooked brown rice

- 2 tablespoons lower-sodium soy sauce

- 1 tablespoon sambal oelek (ground fresh chile paste)

- 1 tablespoon honey

- 2 tablespoons peanut oil, divided

- 10 ounces medium shrimp, peeled and deveined

- 3 large eggs, lightly beaten

- 1½ cups sugar snap peas, diagonally sliced

- ⅓ cup unsalted, dry-roasted peanuts

- ⅛ teaspoon salt

- 3 garlic cloves, crushed

Directions

- Heat rice according to package directions.

- Combine soy sauce, sambal oelek, and honey in a large bowl. Combine 1 teaspoon peanut oil and shrimp in a medium bowl; toss to coat. Heat a wok or large skillet over high heat. Add shrimp to pan, and stir-fry 2 minutes. Add shrimp to soy sauce mixture; toss to coat shrimp. Add 1 teaspoon peanut oil to pan; swirl to coat. Add eggs to pan; cook 45 seconds or until set. Remove eggs from pan; cut into bite-sized pieces.

- Add 1 tablespoon oil to pan; swirl to coat. Add rice; stir-fry 4 minutes. Add rice to shrimp mixture. Add remaining 1 teaspoon oil to pan; swirl to coat. Add sugar snap peas, peanuts, salt, and garlic to pan; stir-fry for 2 minutes or until peanuts begin to brown. Add shrimp mixture and egg to pan, and cook for 2 minutes or until thoroughly heated.

Potato Salad

Total Time: 40 Minutes

Ingredients

- 5 pounds Yukon Gold potatoes or Klondike Goldust potatoes

- 2 cups mayonnaise (your favorite brand)

- 1 cup refrigerated sweet pickle relish

- 2 tablespoons yellow mustard, or 1 part yellow + 1 part dijon

- 1 tablespoon apple cider vinegar

- 1 tablespoon celery seeds

- 1/2 teaspoon paprika

- 4-5 hard boiled eggs, peeled and chopped

- 3 celery stalks, diced

- 1/2 cup sweet onion, diced

- 1 tablespoon fresh chopped dill

- Salt and pepper

Directions

- Cut the potatoes into quarters and place them in a large stockpot. Fill the pot with cold water until it is 1 inch over the top of the potatoes. Set the pot over high heat and bring to a boil. Once boiling, add 1 tablespoon salt and cook the potatoes for 13-15 minutes, until fork tender.

- Meanwhile, in a medium bowl mix the mayonnaise, sweet pickle relish including juices, mustard, apple cider vinegar, celery seeds, paprika, 1 teaspoon salt, and pepper to taste. Stir until smooth. Then chop the eggs, celery, onions, and dill.

- Once the potatoes are very tender, drain off all the water. Remove the loose peels and chop the potatoes into 1/2-inch chunks. It's okay if they are soft and crumbly. Place the potatoes in a large bowl. Gently mix in the dressing until it coats the potatoes well. Then stir in the eggs, celery, onions, and dill. Taste, then salt and pepper as needed. Garnish with fresh dill and paprika.

- Cover the potato salad and refrigerate for at least 4 hours. If you have time to make it ahead, it tastes even better on day two! Keep refrigerated in an airtight container for up to one week.

Egg Salad

Total Time: 25 Minutes

Ingredients

- 6 eggs, room temperature

- ¼ cup red onion, finely diced

- ¼ cup mayonnaise

- 1 tablespoon Dijon mustard

- 2 tablespoons parsley, finely diced

- 2 tablespoons chives, finely diced

- 1 teaspoon lemon juice

- kosher salt and freshly ground black pepper, to taste

Directions

- Bring a pot of water to a boil. Then turn the heat to low so there's no bubbles. Use a skimmer to slowly and gently place the eggs in the pot. Turn the heat back to high and boil the eggs for 12 minutes.

- Transfer the eggs to an ice water bath to stop the cooking process and cool completely (at least 15 minutes).

- Peel the hard-boiled eggs, and slice them up to your preferred level of chunkiness. Add the chopped eggs to a mixing bowl along with the red onion, chives, parsley, mayonnaise, Dijon mustard, lemon juice, salt, and pepper. Stir all of the ingredients together, until well combined.

- Enjoy the egg salad straight from the bowl, or in a sandwich or wrap.

Tomato Salad

Total Time: 20 Minutes

Ingredients

- 2 pints grape tomatoes halved, or 3 cups chopped tomatoes

- ¼ cup red onion thinly sliced

- 1 tablespoon fresh herbs basil, oregano, dill, parsley

- 3 tablespoons olive oil

- 1 tablespoon red wine vinegar

- salt & pepper to taste

- ½ cup bocconcini sliced or diced, optional

Directions

- Place tomatoes, red onion, and bocconcini (if using) in a shallow bowl.

- Drizzle with olive oil and red wine vinegar. Toss to combine.

- Season with salt, pepper, and fresh herbs to taste.

Steak, Beetroot, Horseradish & Warm lentil salad

Total Time: 10 Minutes

Ingredients

- 1 tbsp hot horseradish sauce

- 2 tbsp Greek yogurt

- ½ tsp honey

- 1 lemon, juiced

- 200g fillet steak

- 1½ tbsp cold pressed rapeseed oil

- 2 garlic cloves

- 200g frozen peas

- 250g pouch pre-cooked puy lentils

- 120g runner beans, sliced

- 200g pre-cooked beetroot, cut into wedges

- ½ small pack dill, chopped

- two handfuls rocket

Directions

- Whisk together the horseradish, yogurt and honey. Season and add lemon juice to taste.

- Season the steak on all sides with a little salt and black pepper. Heat 1 tbsp oil in a non-stick frying pan. Add the steak and cook to your liking, 2-3 mins on each side for medium rare. Set aside to rest.

- Put the pan back on the heat, add the remaining oil, lightly crush in the garlic, then tip in the peas, lentils, beans and beetroot. Cook for a few mins, stirring, until the peas and beetroot are warmed through. Remove from the heat, then stir through the remaining lemon juice, dill and rocket.

- Thinly slice the steak. Divide the lentil salad between two plates, nestle in the steak and drizzle over the dressing

Roasted Brussel Sprouts and Sweet Potatoes

Total Time: 30 Minutes

INGREDIENTS

- 1 pound Brussels sprouts trimmed and halved

- 2 medium sweet potatoes about 1 cup, peeled and cubed in ¾-inch pieces)

- 2 tablespoons olive oil or avocado oil

- 1 teaspoon balsamic vinegar or apple cider vinegar

- 1 teaspoon salt

- ½ teaspoon ground black pepper

- 1 teaspoon ground cumin

- 1 teaspoon paprika (sweet)

- ¼ teaspoon cayenne pepper

- 1 teaspoon brown sugar or palm sugar (add 2 teaspoons for sweeter taste)

- ¼ cup dried sweetened cranberries

- ¼ cup toasted pecans or walnuts

- 2 tablespoons finely chopped parsley for garnish

DIRECTIONS

- Trim off the ends of the Brussel sprouts and cut in half. Peel sweet potatoes, cut in half, then cut into cubes, about ¾-inch pieces. Transfer to a large bowl.

- Add salt, pepper, cumin, paprika, and cayenne powder to a small bowl and mix well. Drizzle oil and balsamic vinegar over the vegetables and toss well. Then, evenly sprinkle the spice mix over and toss well to coat the veggies.

Cooking Method 1: Air Fryer

- Preheat air fryer to 450°F. Spread seasoned sweet potatoes and Brussel sprouts in a single layer in the air fryer basket.

- Air fry until tender and browned, about 17-20 minutes, flipping them halfway through. Since air fryer models can vary, check at the 17-minute mark to prevent burning.

Cooking Method 2: Oven

- Preheat oven to 450°F. Spread seasoned sweet potatoes and Brussel sprouts in a single layer on an aluminum foil or parchment-lined baking sheet.

- Place the baking sheet in the middle rack of the oven. Roast until tender and browned, about 17-20 minutes, flipping them halfway through. Since oven temperature varies, check at the 17-minute mark to prevent burning.

Finish & Serve

- Transfer the roasted brussel sprouts and sweet potatoes to a serving bowl and toss with dried cranberries and toasted pecans. Sprinkle finely chopped parsley just before serving.

Tofu Stir Fry

Total Time: 25 Minutes

Ingredients

- 2 (14-ounce) packages extra-firm tofu do not use firm, silken or anything other than extra-firm

- 1 tablespoon canola oil or grapeseed oil

- 3 tablespoons low-sodium soy sauce divided, plus additional to taste

- 3 large garlic cloves minced (about 1 heaping tablespoon)

- 1 small bunch green onions finely chopped, divided

- 1 tablespoon minced fresh ginger

- 1–2 teaspoons fresh chili paste (sambal oelek) or 1/4–1/2 teaspoon red pepper flakes

- 10 ounces baby spinach

- 2 tablespoons toasted sesame seeds

- 2 teaspoons sesame oil

For serving:

- Prepared brown rice see Instant Pot Brown Rice

- Cauliflower rice

- Soba or rice noodles

- Quinoa

Directions

- Wrap each block in a double layer of paper towels and pat dry, pressing down on the tofu lightly to squeeze out excess moisture. Cut the tofu into 3/4-inch cubes.

- In a large nonstick skillet or wok, heat the canola oil over medium-high heat. Once the oil is hot but not smoking, add the tofu (be careful, as the oil will splatter a little bit) and drizzle with 1 tablespoon soy sauce. Sauté, stirring every minute or so until the tofu is nicely colored on all sides and the moisture has cooked off, about 8 to 10 minutes. Don't feel that you need to stir constantly. Sitting for a while on one side is what will allow the tofu to brown. Add the garlic, roughly two-thirds of the green onion, ginger, chili paste, and the remaining 2 tablespoons soy sauce. Stir and cook until fragrant, about 1 minute.

- Add several large handfuls of spinach, stirring as you go so that it wilts and you can fit more in the pan. Once the first addition has wilted, continue to add and wilt the spinach by handfuls, until all of the spinach is added. It will seem like a ridiculous amount at first but will cook down considerably. Stir in the sesame seeds. Stir in the sesame oil. Remove from the heat. Sprinkle the reserved green onions over the top. Serve hot, with brown rice, noodles, or whatever you like, along with a few dashes of additional soy sauce and chili paste or flakes to taste.